Brain Fitness

Maximize Your Brain Power and Memory

Disclaimer and Terms of Use:

Effort has been made to ensure that the information in this book is accurate and complete, however, the author and the publisher do not warrant the accuracy of the information, text and graphics contained within the book due to the rapidly changing nature of science, research, known and unknown facts and internet. The Author and the publisher do not hold any responsibility for errors, omissions or contrary interpretation of the subject matter herein. This book is presented solely for motivational and informational purposes only.

Contents

Introduction

Neuroscientists believed that humans were born with a certain number of neurons that die little by little with age. When a neuron dies, it is lost permanently. However, according to new research, the neurotransmitter dopamine can promote the birth of new neurons in adults. So there is hope after all!

It is a simple fact that the human brain changes as a person ages. Over time, our brain's volume and weight diminishes. As a matter of fact, we lose ten percent of our brain's weight between the ages twenty and ninety; but age is not the only factor that triggers brain shrinkage.

The way we live, what we eat, our habits and every part of our lifestyle are major culprits too. Bad habits including poor diet, lack of exercise, alcohol drinking and smoking as well as health conditions like diabetes are believed to accelerate brain shrinkage according to a study. All these things lead to cardiovascular diseases, which reduce the blood flow to our brains.

The question now is: what are we going to do about it?

Brain Fitness is all about doing the right things and avoiding the wrong ones as much as possible. It is not just enough that we perform activities that encourage the release of dopamine to give birth to new neurons. More importantly, we need a lifestyle change.

Keep this in mind: everything that we do has a huge impact on our overall health. Whether it is a negative or positive effect, it will depend on what we choose. If it is bad for the body, it is more likely worse for the mind. So, don't do anything you will surely regret!

We work our brains out every single day. We use it often and more often than not, we do not even realize how hard our brain works. It is time to give back. Do yourself a favor and make an effort to keep your brain fit and healthy.

This book contains all the basic information you need to maximize your brainpower and keep your memory sharp. Read on and use it wisely!

Chapter 1 – The Key to Staying Sharp

Many individuals are so conscious when it comes to their physique. They spend countless hours planning a healthy diet and doing exercise to make their bodies fit. They cling on to the mantra, "use it or lose it." But this saying does not only apply to muscles in the body. It is also applicable to the neural pathways in the human brain. In which case, we have to pay as much attention to brain fitness as we do physical fitness.

In essence, there are five main cognitive functions that consist inside our brains. These are the following.

1. Memory

2. Language

3. Attention

4. Visual-Spatial Skills and

5. Executive function

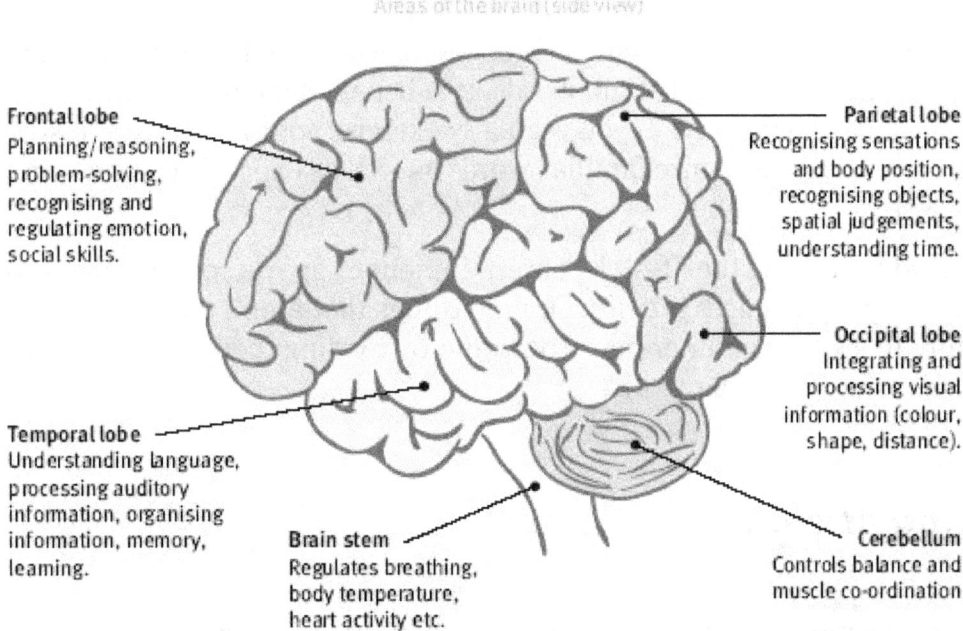

Areas of the brain (side view)

Frontal lobe Planning/reasoning, problem-solving, recognising and regulating emotion, social skills.

Parietal lobe Recognising sensations and body position, recognising objects, spatial judgements, understanding time.

Occipital lobe Integrating and processing visual information (colour, shape, distance).

Temporal lobe Understanding language, processing auditory information, organising information, memory, learning.

Brain stem Regulates breathing, body temperature, heart activity etc.

Cerebellum Controls balance and muscle co-ordination

The truth is, the human brain ages too. The less we use it, the more likely we are to lose it. And like a muscle, it improves with exercise. If you want to be mentally sharp and stay that way, it is crucial that you keep on challenging and stimulating your brain by performing effective exercises that target these 5 main cognitive functions.

Improving Memory

Memory has a huge role to play in all cognitive activities that we do every day, such as reading, mental calculations and reasoning. To have and maintain an excellent memory, you have to train your brain well. Now this may be easier said than done. With already too much on your plate, can you make room for a separate workout?

Improving your memory with exercise does not really involve complex tasks. But you do need to give some time for it and it can be challenging too. For instance, listen to a song you have never heard before and memorize the lyrics. This exercise can help increase your level of acetylcholine, which is the chemical that assists in building the brain as well as in improving memory skills. Or try to get dressed in the dark for a change or brush your teeth using the opposite hand. These things are beneficial in building new links between the different neural connections of your brain.

Enhancing Language Skills

Activities targeted towards enhancing language skills are also helpful in our ability to remember, recognize and understand words. It is beneficial to our vocabulary, grammatical skills and fluency. If you regularly exercise your language skills, you can better and more easily recognize familiar words as well as expand your knowledge of unfamiliar words.

If you are used to reading the lifestyle, entertainment or sports section, challenge your brain by reading the business articles. Or read things that aren't exactly your cup of tea. You are more likely to encounter new words and by reading them in context, it becomes easier for you to understand them.

Improving Attention

This is one of the most important functions that clearly need attention. After all, we use it in almost all of our tasks. If you have excellent attention, you can maintain your concentration even when there are plenty of distractions around you. Good attention also allows you to focus on more than one activity at the same time.

If you want to improve your level of attention, you can try changing up your routine. It is easy to stick with what works, but research says a little change is good especially in enhancing your attention level. So, try something different like reorganizing your desk. The change will push the brain to wake up. The thing is when we get used to doing the same things day in and day out, it becomes a habit and we do it even without actually thinking. It becomes automatic. But as you change things up, your brain will recognize the change and will pay attention once more.

Older individuals have a lower attention span. So as we age, we find it more difficult to push through all the noise and distractions and focus. This also makes us less efficient when it comes to multitasking. But you can achieve efficiency once again by forcing the brain to do several activities at once. For instance, try jogging while listening to an audio book. Combining more than one activity at once works by forcing the brain to do more with the same amount of time.

Enhancing Visual-Spatial Skills

We will be able to act more efficiently in our three dimensional environment if we can analyze visual information better. To exercise this specific cognitive function, try this. Walk in a room and pay attention to the first five items you see as you walk by. As soon as you get out of the room, try to recall these five items and their exact location. Now, this may be too easy. To challenge your brain some more, wait two hours and try recalling again. Can you still remember the five items and their location?

You can try this simple exercise while killing time. Remember to look straight ahead as you walk by. Note the things you see right in front of you as well as those that are visible in your peripheral vision. Then, recall everything that you saw and write them down. Did you remember anything? More than a memory exercise, this activity also forces your brain to pay more attention to your surroundings.

Building up Reasoning Skills

We use logic and reasoning all the time. We do on a regular basis and we often do without even realizing it. You use your logic and reasoning when you make decisions or think about the consequences of these decisions and certain actions. So, how do you exactly enhance your reasoning skills?

You can always join a debate team. But you can also engage in activities that require you to draft a strategy for reaching a desired outcome like in video games. Video games force you to calculate moves to achieve a specific solution in the shortest time possible. Social interaction is also helpful in this regard. So, visit a friend and have a chat. It actually helps in boosting your intellectual performance as you are challenged to come up with responses and consider the possible outcomes.

Both physical and mental exercises are important. And their level of importance increases as we age. We need a conscious effort to build and enhance these cognitive functions. In the succeeding chapters, you will find more ideas for breaking a "mental" sweat and getting your brain into shape.

Chapter 2 – Work Out the Body to Exercise the Mind

There are plenty of activities that you can do to exercise your brain. And when you think about brain exercises, the first thing that comes to mind is probably brain games like crossword puzzles or what have you. You may never think about doing physical exercise to boost your brainpower but you actually should.

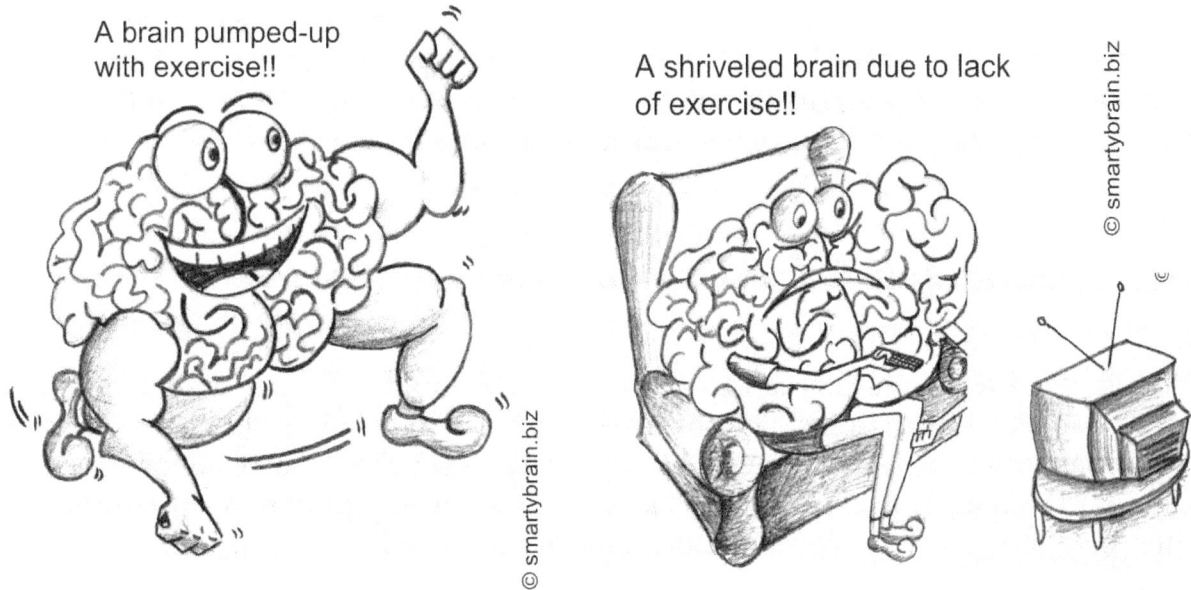

The Annals of Internal Medicine recently published an article that points out the results of a study suggesting that regularly working out for at least 15 minutes a day, three times weekly can help in delaying the onset of Alzheimer's disease. They also reduce the onset of dementia by 32 percent. This study is only one among many that supports the connection between brain fitness and physical exercise.

The fact is that the human brain works like the rest of the muscles in the human body. Now, we are all familiar with the physical benefits of exercise. But did you know that physical exercise also has a positive impact on your brain functions? Scientific research links physical exercise to the reduction of inflammation as it works to stimulate and release new blood vessels in the brain. Why is this important? Inflammation is associated with memory decline but with regular physical exercise, such can be prevented.

As exercises stimulate the generation and help with the survival of new blood vessels in the brain, it also helps lessen your risk of developing vascular dementia, which comes as a result of damaged blood vessels in the brain. Moreover, physical exercise decreases insulin resistance and insulin resistance is known as a major contributor to cognitive decline. It is also one of the leading causes of Alzheimer's disease.

According to the British Journal of Sports Medicine Study, one in 86 women between the ages 70 to 80 suffer from a mild cognitive impairment. This involves a compromise on the hippocampus, which is known as the center of the brain and is responsible for memory and learning. But by spending twice a week for six straight months taking part in aerobic training, this can be prevented. This results to an increase in the hippocampal volume.

Physical exercise does not offer any guarantee of preventing memory related illness altogether. However, research says it does have a positively huge impact on the brain, which should be more than enough to convince you to get on your feet and get fit not only for the sake of your physique but also in the name of brain fitness.

How Does Aerobic Exercises Work the Brain?

Physical exercises, specifically aerobic exercise, positively affect human brain function and they do on multiple fronts. The positive impact of aerobics on the brain ranges from the molecular to the behavioral level. A study conducted by the Department of Exercise Science at the University of Georgia, demonstrates that working out even for only 20 minutes improves memory functions and information processing.

Aerobic exercises increase your heart rate. And as the heart rate increases, more oxygen is pumped into the brain. Physical workouts also encourage the release of various hormones. These hormones are crucial in the assisting and creating a nourishing environment ideal for stimulating brain cell growth.

Aerobic exercises also work by stimulating the growth of new connections between brain cells in different cortical areas of the brain. And therefore, it builds up brain plasticity. Researchers from UCLA found that exercise helps expand growth factors in the human brain. As a result, the brain finds it easier to build new neuronal connections.

But exercise does not only affect the brain in the molecular front. It also has a huge impact on the behavioral front. As it turns out, exercise provides the same benefits as anti-depressants in individuals taking such medicines. Physical workout gives individuals what is known as the "runner's high." It is known to reduce stress hormone levels in the body. According to a study from Stockholm, running is also linked to the stimulation of more cell growth in the hippocampus or that area of the human brain associated with memory and learning.

Taking it Double Time: A Combination of Mental and Physical Exercise is the Best

Physical exercises alone provide huge and positive benefits to brain function. But you maximize its benefits further as you combine it with brain training. This shall significantly increase cognitive functions.

While jogging, running and cycling does provide benefits to the brain, there are other exercises that offer a higher impact on cognitive functioning. These exercises include those that give both mental and physical demands like ballroom dancing.

Your brain benefits from a more enhanced cognitive function in this kind of activity rather than engaging in physical or mental tasks alone. In which case, the best exercises for brain health are those that involve the different parts of the brain, such as those responsible for strategy, rhythm and coordination.

How to Choose the Right Physical Exercise

We have zeroed in on aerobic exercise being one of the best workouts for both the body and brain. Basically, it acts like a "first aid kit," repairing damaged brain cells and works to improve brain function. But there are more physical exercises that do your brain some good too.

The general rule here is that anything that works great for the heart is also good for the brain. So, when choosing an exercise, opt for those that target the heart.

As mentioned above, it is also wise to choose physical workouts that involve both the mind and body. While it is important to sweat it out, you should also think about maximizing the impact of the workout for your cognitive function. As much as possible, choose those that require coordination and work out the heart as well. So, try taking a dance class.

If you would like a more hard-core exercise in the gym, try circuit training. Such routines do not only pump up your heart rate. They also improve your concentration level as you are forced to constantly redirect your attention from one exercise to another.

Moreover, it is not just a matter of choosing the right form of physical exercise. It is also important to choose the right time to work out. Ideally, exercise should be performed first thing in the morning or before you head to work. This helps increase brain activity. Working out in the morning also prepares you to take on the mental stresses you may encounter throughout the day. It also helps in enhancing your ability to retain new information as well as allow you to better manage complex situations.

Now, what if you feel tired and mentally worn out in the middle of the day? Try some jumping jacks. It will not only make you more alert. It will also help reboot your brain so you can focus better.

Chapter 3 – Eat Brain Foods

The human brain is a powerful organic machine. It is responsible for controlling our thoughts, sensations and movements. At the same time, it calculates and reacts instantaneously.

The human brain is capable of holding and performing thousands of complex functions including hormone balance, blood flow, circadian rhythm, unconscious activity and breathing among many others. Our brains are constantly at work, and it continues to work even when our bodies rest.

With all the functions and responsibilities, the brain understandably requires plenty of energy. While it only weighs about 2 percent of the total body weight, the human brain consumes over 20 percent of our calorie intake. Fifty percent of the energy the brain gets is used for sending bioelectrical messages through the neurons and various parts of the body. It is simply amazing!

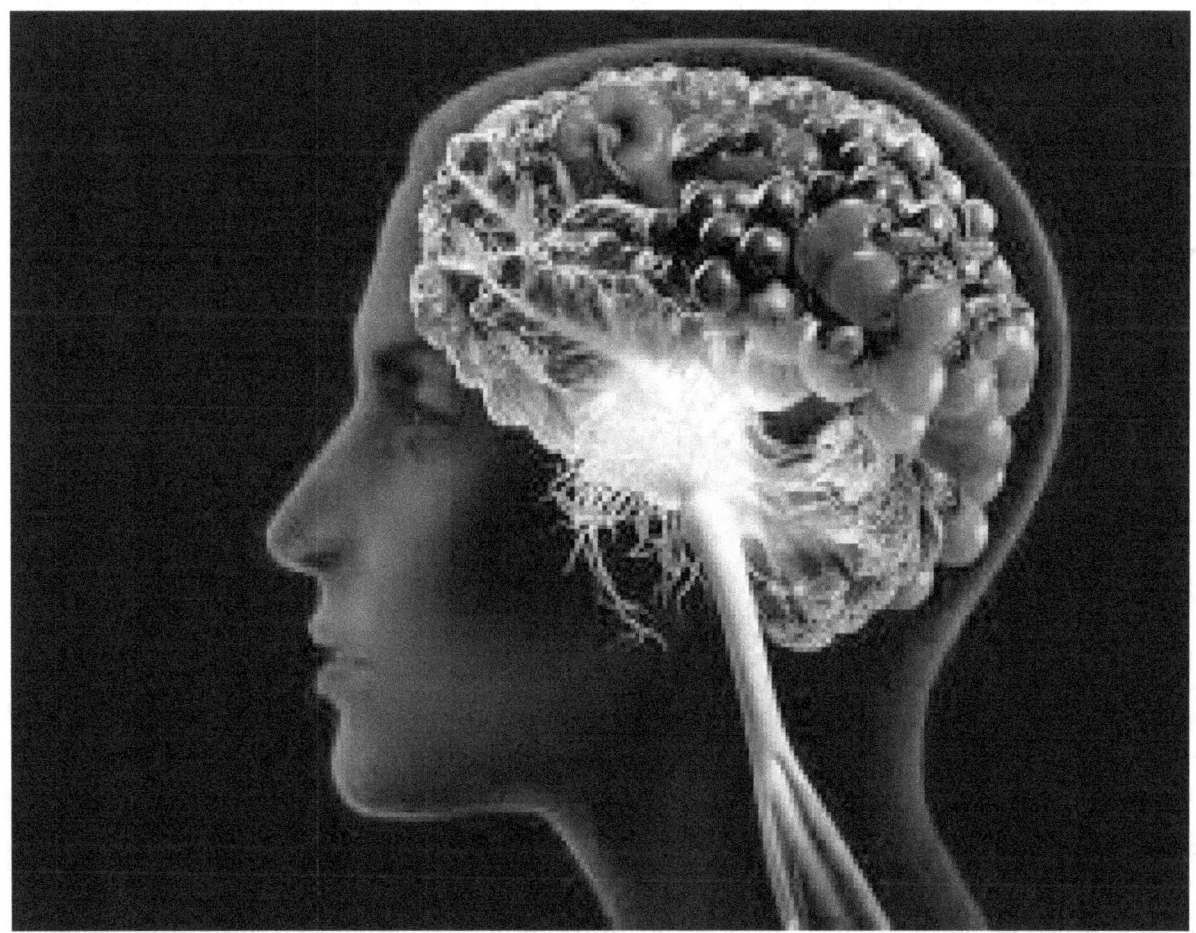

Whatever you eat will affect your body. This is why it is important to be conscious about the things you put into your mouth. In fact, the foods you eat also affect your mood. They also affect the brain's energy as well as the memory. Food also has an impact on the way you handle stress and manage complex tasks.

The Brain Needs Sugar

The human brain demands a load of glucose, so it can keep on running. Because the neurons do not keep a stock of glucose, they tend to be constantly hungry, needy and greedy. Glucose is obtained from carbohydrate-rich foods like grains, fruits and vegetables. But just because the brain requires sugar to function, it does not necessarily mean you must feed it with junk food.

The truth is consuming foods with refined sugars, such as high fructose corn syrup and table sugar, are strongly discouraged. They are not safe options because they will cause sugar spikes. In fact, instead of helping out, they end up causing more damage to your body and brain cells.

Rather than feeding the brain, junk foods actually starve the hungry neurons. As a result, the brain is forced to steal glucose from the fluids nearby. And when the supply runs out, the neurons become sluggish. Consequently, your concentration level and memory suffers too. When this happens often, that is a repeated up and down on glucose supply, the neurons become damaged.

Other Things the Brain Uses

In addition to glucose, the brain uses other nutrients. As a matter of fact, 60 percent of the brain is made of fat. When the body is low in fat, you run the risk of suffering from depression dementia and Alzheimer's disease.

While the brain and body requires fat, you don't just eat any kind of fat. It is crucial that you pick out the healthy ones. Choose those that are found in nuts, algae, seeds, avocados and coconut. These foods offer essential omega 3 fatty acids and balance out omega 6.

Saturated fats may also be required, but you should always have some in moderation. Coconut oil, in particular, is helpful in increasing the level of good cholesterol. It is also beneficial for weight loss. And more importantly, it plays a huge role in fighting off brain degeneration and disorders.

What you should avoid altogether are trans fats. They are commonly found in hydrogenated vegetable oils. Rather than being helpful, they are extremely harmful. They increase bad cholesterol level. In addition, trans fats also cause damage to the heart and brain. If you want to feed your brain, you should stick to plant-based foods that enhance brain function, improve memory and mood.

Top Brain Foods to Eat

To get an idea of the foods you should be eating, below is a list of the best brain foods that promote overall brain fitness.

Avocado

Rich in omega3 and omega 6 essential fatty acids and monounsaturated fats, avocados help in increasing the blood flow to the brain. They also work at lowering bad cholesterol level as well as assist in the proper absorption of antioxidants. Moreover, avocados bring in a load of vitamin E and other antioxidants that serve to protect your brain and body from damages done by free radicals.

Beans and Legumes

These foods provide the brain and body with complex carbohydrates. Fiber and complex carbohydrates work hand in hand in slowing down absorption. In effect, sugar spikes are prevented. The brain benefits from a steady supply of glucose. Also rich in folate, beans and legumes are essential to optimum brain function.

Blueberries

Known as an antioxidant powerhouse, blueberries have the ability to protect the brain from stress and oxidative damage, which often cause premature aging, dementia and Alzheimer's. The flavonoids that blueberries contain also enhance the communication between neurons. They enhance learning ability, improve memory and build up other cognitive functions such as decision making, reasoning and verbal comprehension among others. Aside from blueberries, dark berries including acai, goji berries and blackberries are excellent brain foods as well.

Broccoli

High in vitamins B, C and K, beta-carotene, calcium, fiber and iron, broccoli is considered a super food. The nutrients it contains serve to protect the brain and body against free radicals. They also aid in circulation and the elimination of heavy metals that cause damage to the brain.

Coldwater Fish

This includes sardines, salmon, mackerel, trout, tuna and sardines. They are good for the brain because they are rich in omega-3 fatty acids, which are among the best brain foods. Coldwater fish are particularly rich in docosahexaenonic acid or DHA, which offer the most brain benefits.

These fishes offer neuroprotection that can extend throughout your lifespan. In fact, it aids in the promotion of healthy brain to newborns and enhance cognitive function in adults. A specific study suggests that mothers who consume enough amount of DHA from their diets are more likely to have smart kids. Salmon, sardines and shrimp also contain vitamin B12, which is crucial in neuroprotection as well as in building up cognitive health.

In 2005, the Archives of Neurology published a study that demonstrated fish benefits to brain health. According to the study, older people who consumed fish at least once a week experience about 10 percent slower decline on their cognitive tests. Another study demonstrated that men and women over 65 who ate fish weekly lower their risk of Alzheimer's by 60 percent.

Coconut Oil

An excellent source of medium chain triglycerides, coconut oil provides the body with the energy it requires to function properly. This means, coconut oil also feeds the brain enough glucose. An anti-inflammatory food, coconut oil is believed to prevent dementia and Alzheimer's disease.

Chia

An excellent source of fiber and omega 3 fatty acids, chia is another great brain food you should not miss out on. These seeds help in controlling blood glucose levels. They are also anti-inflammatory. And they promote proper hydration.

Dark Chocolate

Rich in flavonols, dark chocolate enhances blood vessel function. In turn, this builds up memory and other cognitive functions. Filled with antioxidants, chocolate helps ease the mood and pain.

Eggs

Have eggs for breakfast! They are rich in Choline, which is believed to be essential in long-term memory development. This specific nutrient also plays a major role in the neurotransmitter acetylcholine that is important for healthy neurotransmission. According to research studies, the Choline found in eggs may be able to help in the recovery of individuals suffering from learning memory disorders. As a matter of fact, eggs can also possibly improve psychic function specifically for people with Alzheimer's disease and senile dementia. In addition to its Choline content, the yolks are also filled with omega 3 essential fatty acids, which also contribute to brain health.

Nuts

Almonds and walnuts specifically are excellent for the brain and the entire nervous system. These nuts also contain omega 3 and 6 fatty acids, vitamins B6 and E. These nutrients play a critical role in protecting the brain against free radical damage as well as in empowering the brain. To make nuts healthier, try soaking them overnight or for at least 8 hours before consuming them so you maximize their brain benefits.

Quinoa

This is another brain food that contains complex carbohydrates and fibers, which are essential in regulating blood sugar level and at the same time, provide glucose for the brain. Rich in iron and B vitamins, quinoa keeps the blood oxygenated, protects the blood vessels and improves mood. It is recommended that you soak quinoa overnight before cooking.

Red Cabbage

This food is excellent for both the heart and brain due to its polyphenol content. It also contains glucosinolates, which are believed to fight cancer.

Rosemary

Essential in improving memory and cognitive function, rosemary does more than simply make your meals smell good. Rosemary is known to help in improving the flow of blood to the brain.

Spinach

Popeye seems to know a lot about spinach. Other than providing a boost of strength, these leafy greens prevent tumor growth, DNA damage and cancer cell growth. It is also known to slow down the effects of brain aging and delay the onset of dementia.

Sunflower Seeds

Contains omega fatty acids, protein and B vitamins, sunflower seeds provide the body with essential nutrients. They are also rich in tryptophan, which is converted to serotonin, known to improve mood and fight off depression. What's even healthier than the seeds are the sunflower sprouts and micro greens?

Tomatoes

Rich in lycopene, tomatoes are linked to the prevention of dementia as well as in promoting balanced mood.

Whole Grains

These grains are important in protecting both the heart and brain from blood sugar fluctuations because of their fiber, omega 3 and complex carbohydrate content. Also filled with B vitamins, whole grains encourage healthy blood flow to the brain. To release the nutrients in whole grains, make sure to soak, ferment, sprout or grow them as micro greens. Such also helps in minimizing its anti-nutrients content.

Other excellent brain foods include asparagus, bananas, chicken, cinnamon, cucumber, flaxseeds, lamb, lentils, milk, oats, onions, pomegranate, sage, seaweed, sesame seeds, sweet potatoes, turmeric, watermelon, winter squash and the like. As with physical exercise, the rule of thumb in food is that anything that is beneficial to the heart and promotes proper circulation is extremely helpful to brain function as well. So eat well and eat right to boost your brainpower!

Here's a brain recipe you should try. It is meant to enhance your focus and concentration level as well as provide you with a long lasting energy throughout the day.

Ingredients:

1. Twenty ounces of filtered water

2. Six ounces of organic blueberries

3. Two tablespoons of hemp seeds

4. One tablespoon of coconut oil

5. One tablespoon of Spirulina powder

6. One tablespoon of raw cacao powder

7. One tablespoon of organic and raw honey

Pour the water in the blender, and then toss everything else in. Blend until smooth and enjoy its brain boosting power!

Chapter 4 – Play Brain Games

As mentioned earlier, as your body needs a work out, your brain needs a dose of exercise as well. Here are some mental games you can play and have fun while you are at it!

Crosswords

According to research, crossword puzzles help in enhancing a specific brain function. That is fluency. It enhances your word finding ability. Fluency is that brain function that is based on language and speech.

The 1960 Season

Across

1. Cy Young Award winner
3. Only active member of the 3,000 hit club in 1960
6. Yankee pitcher who threw two complete game World Series shutouts
8. AL 1959 HR leader traded for Kuenn, the batting champ
10. Wrote 'Fear Strikes Out'
11. Star whose glove was stolen prior to the first 1960 All Star game
12. Pitched a no-hitter in first start after being traded to Cubs
17. Pitcher who led NL in appearances
19. Cardinal manager
20. Winningest lefty pitcher in history
21. Yankee pitcher who gave up Maz's famous homer
22. Led NL in doubles

Down

2. Baseball legend who ended his career with his 521 homers
3. AL's largest seating capacity stadium
4. Detroit pitcher with most complete games
5. Reds pitcher 'Calvin Coolidge Julius Caesar Tuskahoma...'
7. Yankee pitcher who was first choice in December expansion draft
9. Yankee sent to the A's for Roger Maris
11. Giant HOF pitching star signed for $500
13. Detroit manager 'traded' for Indians manager Joe Gordon
14. "Beat'em..." was Pirate fight song
15. NL Home Run leader
16. Pirate catcher with key home run in World Series game 7
17. Led AL in triples
18. Slugger who said, "I'm no home-run hitter."

Although complex crosswords can be frustrating, you have to keep your mind challenged. Simple crosswords that are not challenging enough won't do much for your brain. Choose those that will force your brain to work to the next level.

Jigsaw Puzzles

Try a jigsaw puzzle consisting of no less than 500 pieces. While they may seem mundane, jigsaw puzzles can make a difference to how your brain works.

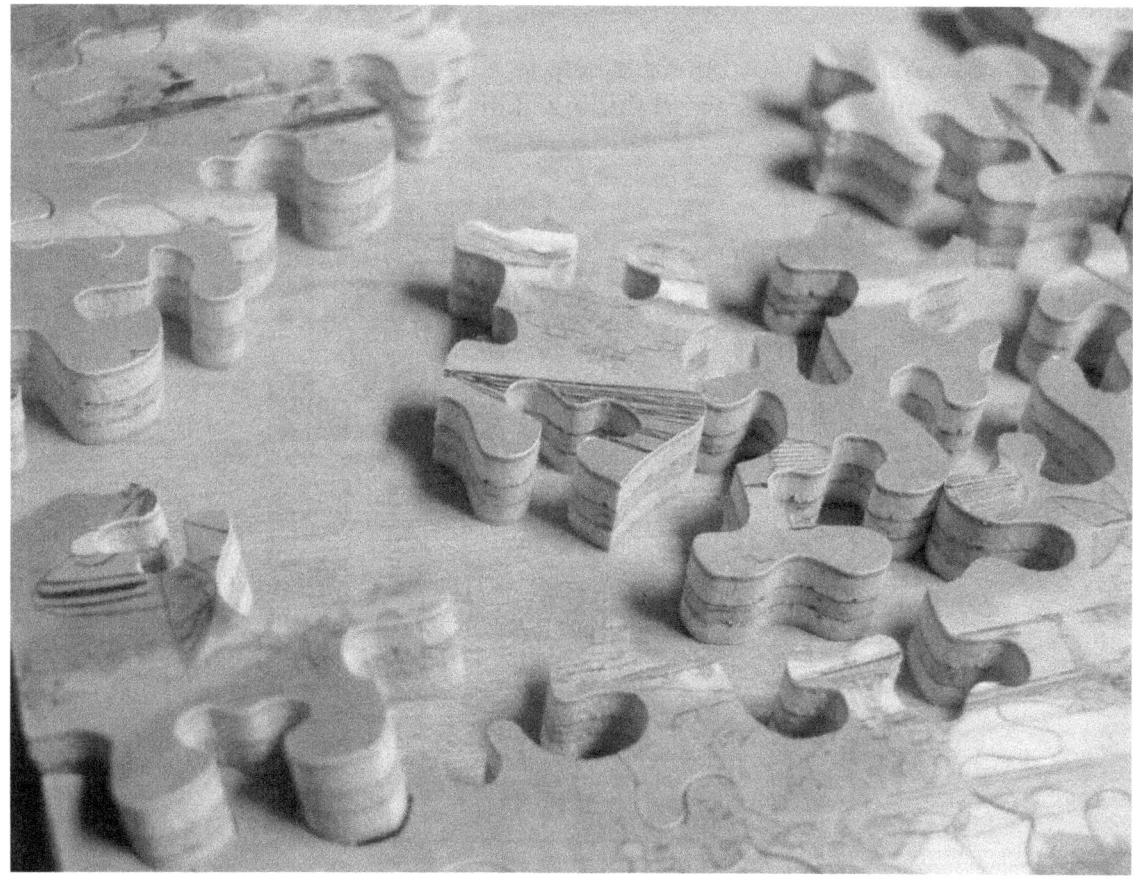

It takes a fine visual judgment for you to be able to complete one. You have to figure out where each piece belongs. That means you have to mentally rotate the pieces, work with your hands to manipulate them. It also requires the brain to constantly shift attention and focus from one piece to another until you complete the big picture. And the best part is, it feels rewarding once you have completed it.

Sudoku

A numbers game that has widespread popularity, Sudoku requires you to fill the blank boxes provided in the puzzle based on certain specific rules. Why would you get on this game?

	9							
	5							
	1							
4	3	9	1	6	8	2	7	5
	7							
	8							
	6		7	4	3			
	4		9	2	1			
	2		5	8	6			

For one, Sudoku helps improve memory. This brain game demands the use of both logic and memory. You need to keep the numbers in mind. At the same time, you have to use logic to figure out what number to put into each blank box. By keeping your logical thinking process exercised in solving the Sudoku puzzle, you also get to improve your number skills.

This numbers game is also beneficial to improving your concentration level as Sudoku demands strategic thinking for problem solving. You need to concentrate on the filling out each blank piece. Moreover, this brain game increases your sense of time. There is a sense of urgency. In which case, your ability to learn and solve it quickly is improved. Sudoku teaches you how to make a decision and how to be decisive in taking action.

Finally, at the end of the game, you will not only feel relief. Having completed a challenging game gives you a sense of accomplishment.

Stroop Test or Stroop Effect

This brainteaser is designed to put your executive attention capacity to test. Here's how it works: quickly say the colors aloud. Do not simply read the word. Rather, say the color that you actually see in each word.

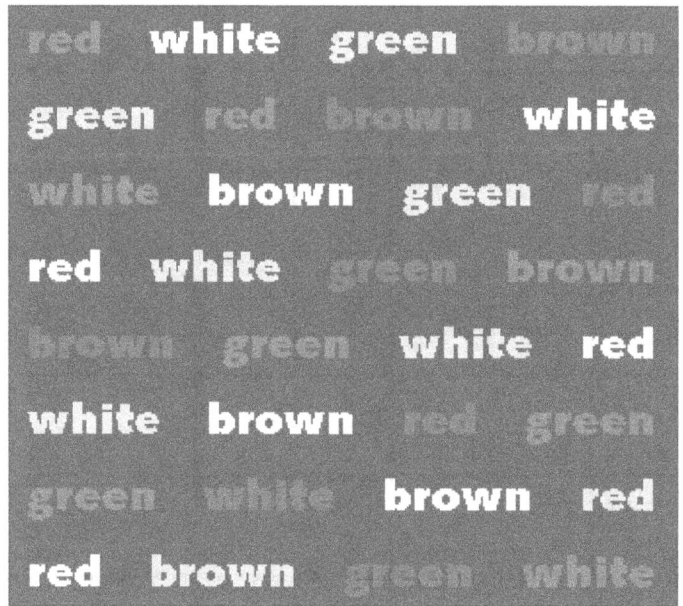

This test used commonly used in neuropsychological evaluations to assess mental flexibility and vitality. In order to perform well, you must pay keen attention and you should also practice self-regulation skills.

3, 6, 7

Here's something that the military has been using for years. This brainteaser is designed to challenge the frontal lobe, which is responsible for attention and memory, along with the parietal lobe, which is in charge of visual interpretation.

Here's what to do: Look at the series of numbers below. Count how many times the number "6" appears. Then, count how many times the numbers "3" and "7" appears.

```
12344678899746746578658765765 35765736254326573465784365783 42
273218858273582745672468734382 8 7672878682768723682376783768267
264764882317834643276487677465 3 7436574386581483627868653873465
```

Now you realize just how challenging this is. As used by the military, this brain exercise can help improve your attention level.

Days and Letters Exercise

This brainteaser comes from Dr. Harriet Vines, who is a retired college professor and experienced author. This brainteaser is meant to put your working memory and attention to work.

1. Speak the days of the week, but say it backwards. Then, say them in alphabetical order.

2. Now, say the months of the year and do so in alphabetical order. That sounds easy enough. Then, try to say them backwards. It is still pretty much doable. Now, say them again backwards in alphabetical order.

3. Calculate the sum of your birth date (mm/dd/yyyy). Next, find the sum of your friends' and family's birth date.

4. Identify two objects that start with every letter in your full name. Let's make it more challenging. This time, name five objects. Make sure you identify different items for every letter.

5. Look around you. In two minutes, you should find and identify five red items that fit right into your pocket and five blue items that are too big for your pocket.

Visual Illusions

This can be a whole lot of fun. But they are not just all about having fun. Here's how it works in the brain.

You see the human brain consists of two hemispheres that are divided into four separate lobes with each lobe in charge of different functions. For example, our frontal cortex is in control of planning and decision-making while the temporal lobe is responsible for memory and language. The parietal lobe on the other hand, works spatial skills. And the occipital lobe is responsible for vision.

Researchers have devoted years studying how the visual system reads colors, shapes, sizes and other elements. And part of the study is to find out whether or not the visual system can be tricked and to check how the brain responds to visual illusions.

1. Look at the squares. Then, look at the squares within the squares. Do you see the same color in the blue and yellow squares?

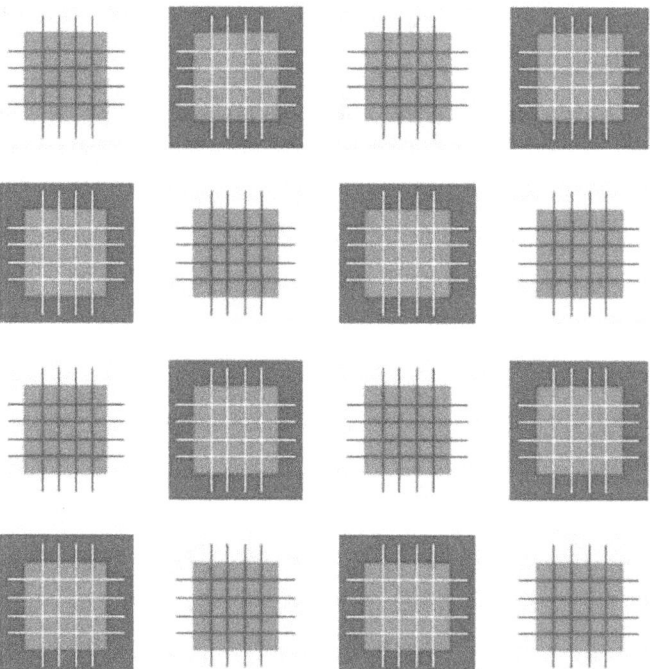

2. Take a good look at the circles. Are they fixed or are they moving?

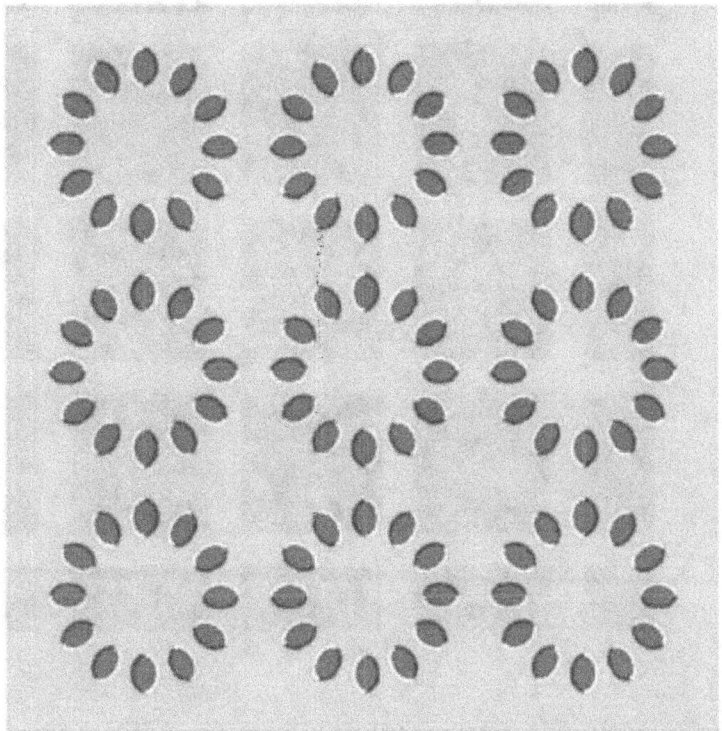

3. This is called the Hermann Grid. How many colors do you recognize in this figure?

4. Try to focus on the two horizontal lines. Are they of the same length or is one longer than the other?

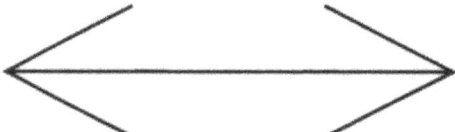

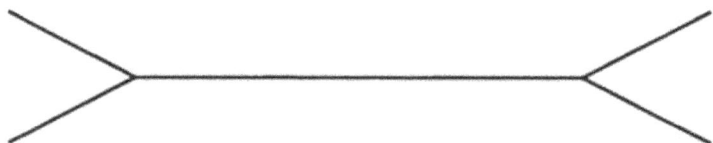

5. Looks familiar? Does this man's face look normal to you?

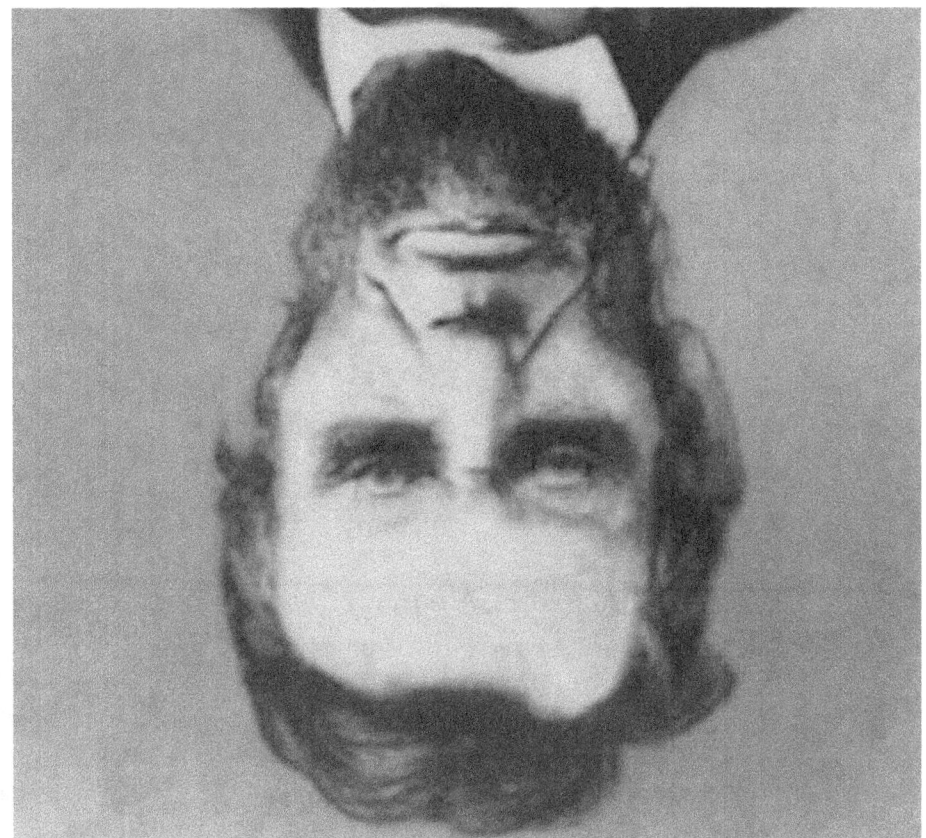

6. This elephant looks normal enough. Now pay attention to its legs? How many do you see?

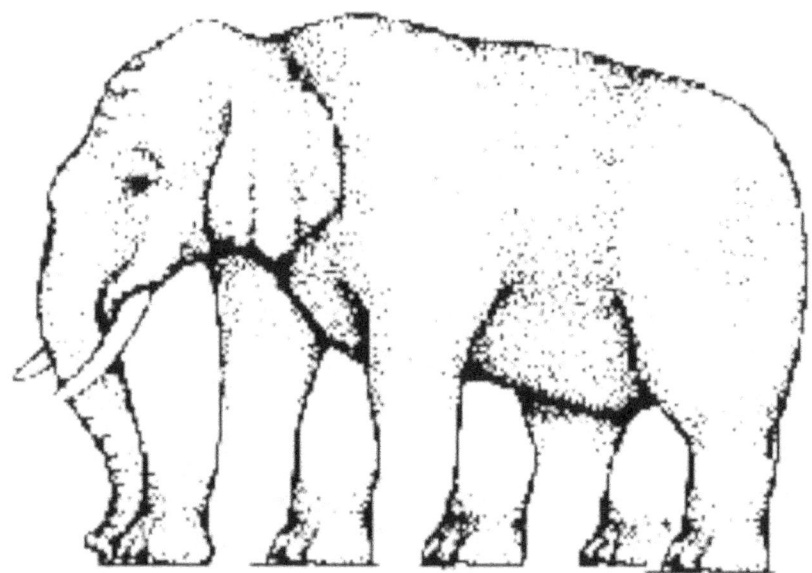

7. Pay attention to the horizontal lines. Are they straight or do they look crooked?

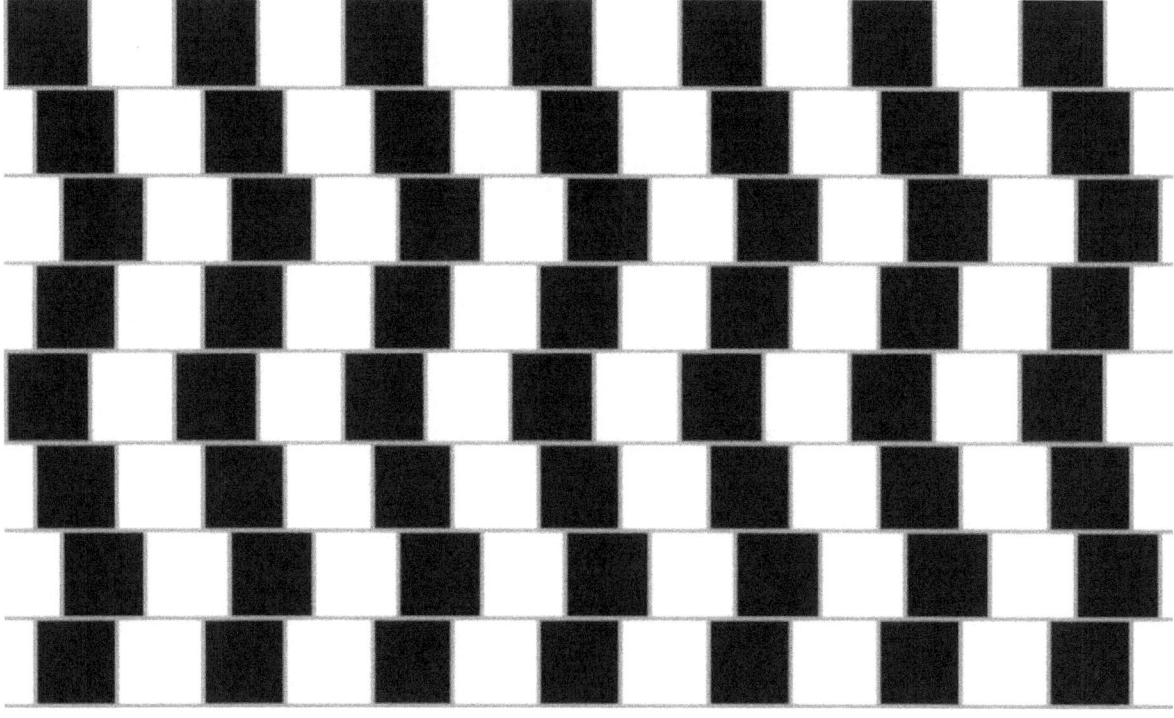

8. Try to focus on the orange circles in the middle of the blue ones. Are the orange circles of the same size? Or is one bigger than the other?

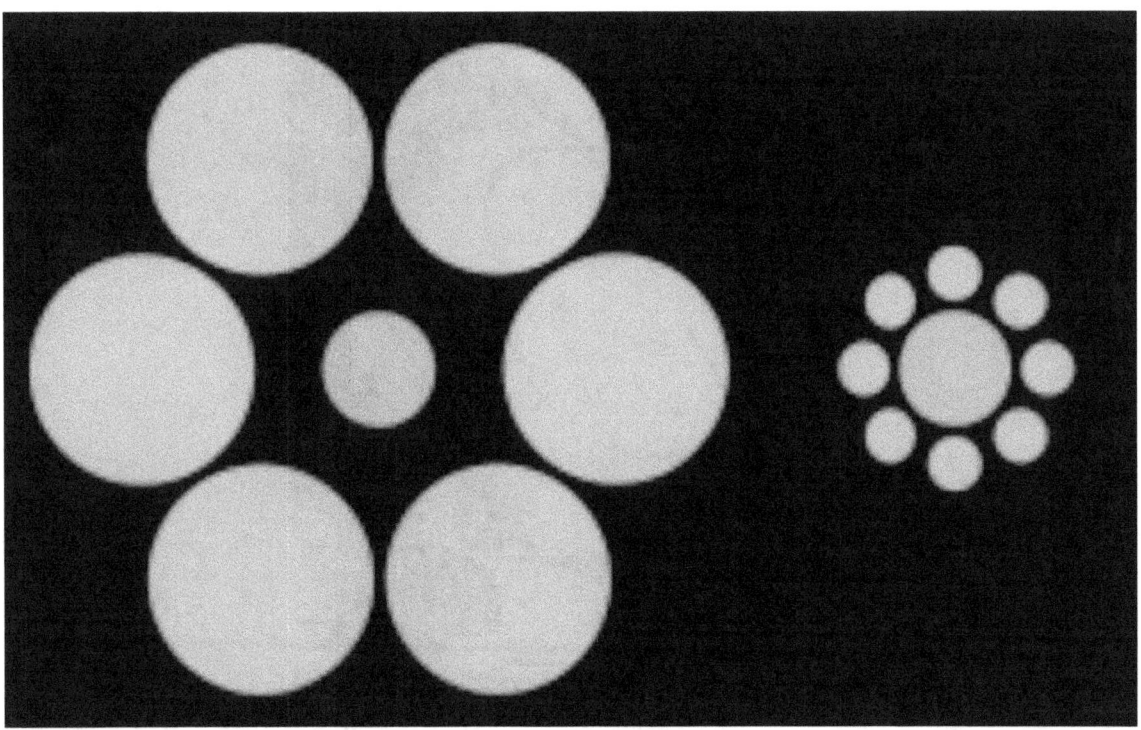

9. Find the baby in this picture.

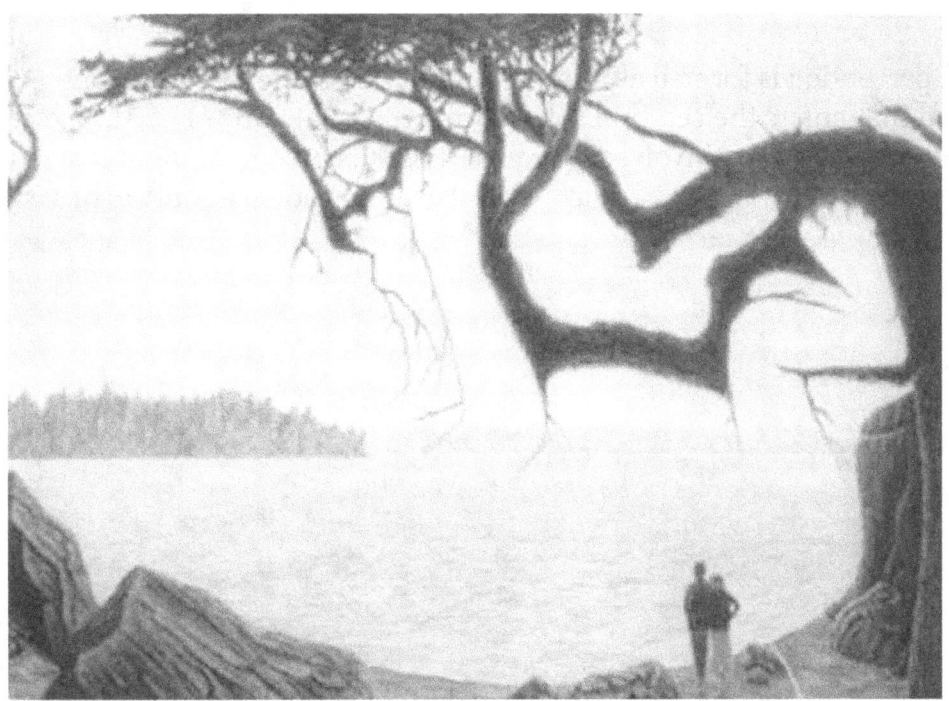

10. What do you see in this picture?

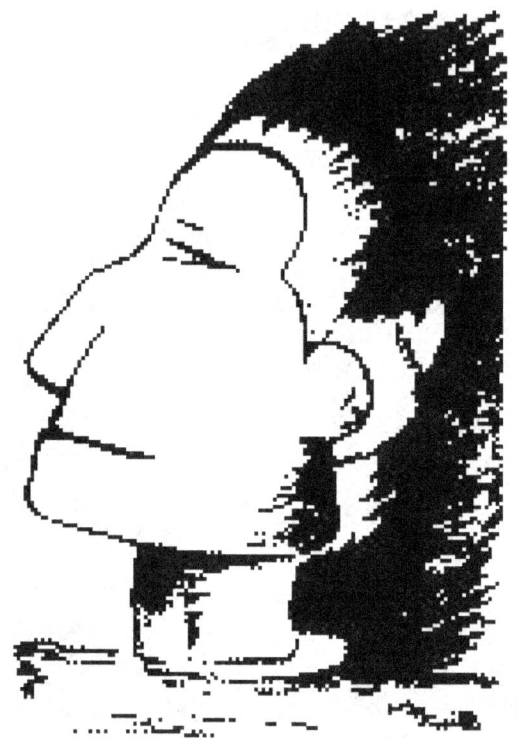

Our visual perception is formed as a result of the brain's interpretation of the visual information that enters the cerebral cortex through visual pathways. More often than not, the mind becomes too involved in translating the perceptual input instead of passively recording it. This is why we make mistakes. It is known as optical or visual illusions.

Chapter 5 – Try Meditation

In recent years, there has been an explosion of scientific research pointing out the extraordinary health benefits of meditation. And there is one particular benefit that catches a lot of attention. That is the neuroscience findings. According to research studies, the brain can be sculpted in the same way as muscles can be toned and built. And such can be done through meditation.

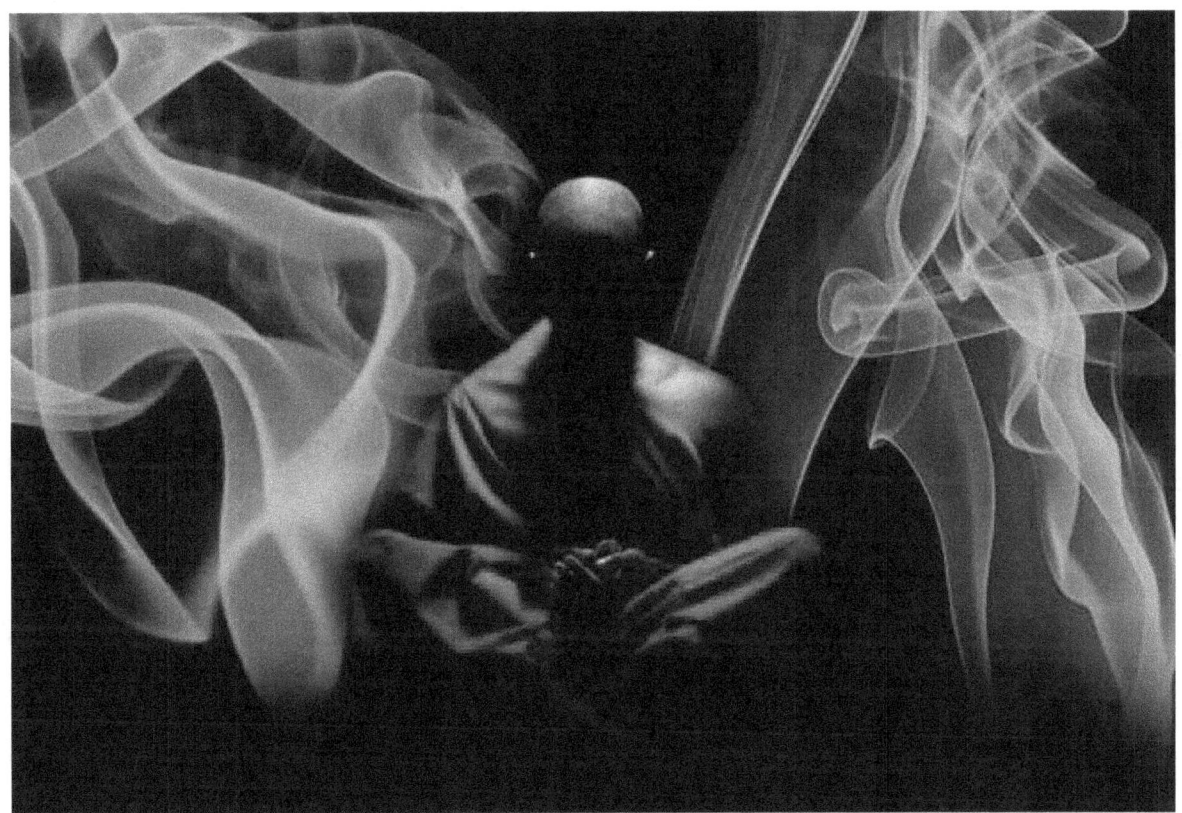

Apparently, we can do something about our resilience, well-being and impulse control. It is not set from birth after all. You and I can do a neurosurgery. We have the capacity to rewire our brains. But how does meditation exactly boost brainpower?

Meditation Helps Build Resilience

When the researchers from the University of Wisconsin-Madison performed a scan on the Tibetan monks' brains, they have found a connection between resilience and meditation. Researchers focused on the region of the brain that is responsible for emotions and the corresponding emotional memories. From their findings, they have come to the conclusion that with the help of meditation, we can recover faster and easier from stress and trauma.

Meditation Thickens the Gray Matter

Critics questioned the findings of researchers from the University of Wisconsin-Madison citing that the brains of Tibetan monks cannot be compared to the brains of the rest of the population. It may be true. But the next study will shock you.

Researchers at Harvard conducted an MRI study. They have gathered people who had no previous experience with meditation. These people were given an eight-week meditation course. After the meditation course, the MRI study was conducted. And the results showed a thicker gray matter specifically in the brain regions that are linked to compassion and self-awareness. Moreover, the area of the brain associated with stress literally shrank.

Meditation Helps Silence the Voices in Our Heads

Yale conducted a study that is focused on the brain region also known as "default mode network." This part of the brain becomes active as we get too involved and lost in our own thoughts, pondering about the past, worrying about the future or just obsessing about our personal issues.

According to the research findings, people who meditated actually deactivated this particular brain region while they are in the process of meditation and even after the session. This could mean meditation can help create an entirely new and different default mode, a more positive one that is.

Meditation Can Help Improve Focus

Meditation teaches us to let go of thoughts and concentrate on breathing. It teaches us to relax and be in control not letting distractions get in the way. That is exactly what the UC Santa Barbara researchers found. According to the scientists, meditation is quite helpful in reducing the tendency of the mind to wander off. And meditation helped students perform much better on their Graduate Record Exam.

Meditation Teaches Us to Manage Stress Better

A study from the University of Miami looked into three groups of extremely stressed out people. The first group involved incarcerated youth. The second consisted of college students and the third included Marines who are about to be sent overseas. Each group showed just how helpful meditation can be even if performed in short bursts. A few minutes of daily meditation protected these people from stress-related degradation of specific brain functions specifically those associated with short-term memory and attention.

Meditation for Beginners

There is a couple of things you should keep in mind before, after and during a meditation session. Here are a couple of guidelines to perform meditation on your own.

1. Prepare yourself well before meditation. You should stay alert and therefore consuming alcoholic drinks, non-prescription drugs and smoking are prohibited at least 24 hours before the session.

2. Do not meditate on an empty stomach. But you should not meditate right after meals either. Wait at least 3 hours after a meal before you start a session.

3. Wear comfortable clothing. Choose loose clothing. Ideally, your shoes should be removed too.

4. Choose a quiet spot where you will not be disturbed.

5. Put away your mobile phone or any kind of distractions.

6. Make your meditation spot pleasant. Although not required, it may help you a bit to light up scented candle or incense or put up flowers around. You just need to make sure these pleasantries are helpful. Otherwise, do away with them.

7. Dim the lights. Meditating in complete darkness is not recommended as that may only make you fall asleep. Meditating under bright lights will distract you too. This is why it may be helpful to light a candle instead or simply dim the lights.

8. Sit comfortably. You can use a straight-backed chair or put up some cushions to support your head and back. But if you have chosen an outdoor spot for meditation, you can use the trunk of a tree or a wall for back support. Remember that you will be in this position for 10 minutes or so. It is important that you are comfortable. Any kind of discomfort will only distract you.

9. Once you've found your comfortable spot and position, stay still and quiet.

10. Close your eyes and focus on your breathing. Breathe in deeply and breathe out slowly. Empty your thoughts and focus on how your chest expands every time you inhale and how it contracts every time you exhale. Visualize the air

entering your nose, passing through your throat, chest and belly. Notice how freely it flows in and out.

11. Create a mantra. This can be any sound or phrase you make up to assist the meditation process. Mantras can make a difference and contribute further to the spiritual, transformational and vibrational effects of meditation. You can either speak it out loud or whisper silently. Say it at each breath. You can use the "ooohhhmmmm" sound or simply say, "I am breathing in, I am breathing out."

12. Calm the mind. Free your mind of everything else. Your focus should be on your breathing and on the mantra. Imagine how everything that stresses you out and all the negativity being released as you exhale, or how you welcome positive energy at every time you inhale.

13. To end the session, slowly bring your consciousness back to your surroundings. Acknowledge where you are. Slowly and gently move your toes and fingers. Move a little by little then, open your eyes. Take your time before getting up.

There is no exact set time for meditation. But for beginners, 5 to 15 minutes may be enough for a start. Practice daily and practice often.

Chapter 6 – Sleep Well

Sleep allows our physical bodies to regenerate. But sleep is also critical for gaining new mental insights. It also works to enhance our creativity so we can work a solution around tough problems. Sleep is said to reset the brain. So, when we wake up, we earn a different perspective and look at problems differently.

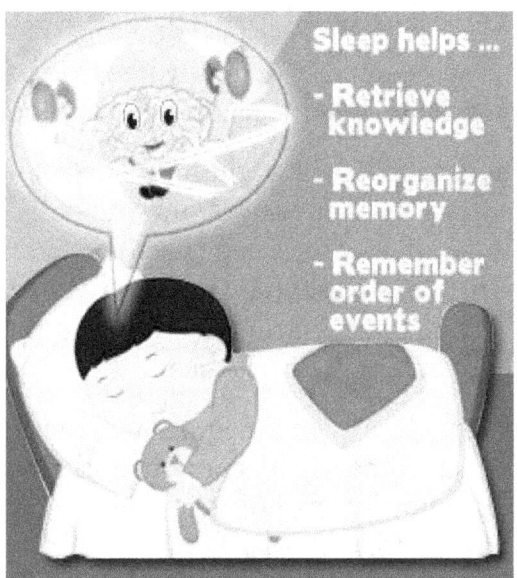

According to a research study from Harvard, individuals are 33 percent more likely to create new connections between and among distantly related concepts or ideas after getting some sleep. However, only a few of us realize just how important sleep is and how much it can help improve our performance.

Sleep is also crucial for memory. It also has a positive impact on your performance, especially when it comes to challenging tasks. An adequate amount of sleep at night can make you think clearly the following day.

Plasticity or the process of growth is thought to trigger the brain's ability to control behavior as well as learning and memory. The process of growth occurs as neurons are fired up by information and events from the environment. Sleep or the lack thereof however, tend to change the reaction of some genes and gene products that may be crucial in synaptic plasticity. In other words, sleep builds up and strengthens synaptic connections. Likewise, these connections are weakened when you are sleep deprived.

Even short naps are quite beneficial. Research shows that babies who take naps between testing and learning sessions experience an enhanced ability to recognize patterns with new pieces of information they are presented. This suggests an important change in their memories. This also contributes significantly to the infant's cognitive development.

Naps are helpful, even among adults. For instance, taking a mid-day nap is believed to considerably increase as well as restore brainpower. So do not fight it. Shut your eyes.

How Much Sleep Do You Need?

There is no question about it. A person cannot go far without getting some serious shuteye. Otherwise, you will not be able to function properly. As a matter of fact, your brain activity is affected and changed when you do not get enough sleep. It turns into something similar as experienced by those with psychiatric disorders.

Now, the question is: how much sleep do you really need? Is a five or six hour sleep at night long enough? Or do you really need to sleep eight to nine hours?

Generally speaking, people require at least eight hours of sleep a night. This notion, however, is based from the practice of our ancestors who had about nine hours of sleep each night. But the eight-hour window for sleep is actually a myth, according to Professor Jim Horne from the Sleep Research Centre. Just because our ancestors slept nine hours every night, it does not necessarily mean we should too. We do not have to pattern our sleeping time based from their practice.

While children between the ages 8 to 17 may require more sleeping time, adults can function with much less. In fact, some adults perform at their peak even with just six to seven hours of night sleep. By allotting six hours for sleeping time, you may get enough rest to make you think clearly the following day.

Sleeping more or less than enough can cause serious problems. For instance, in a research study conducted by the National Institutes of Health, people who had nine or more hours of sleep each night are nearly twice more likely to suffer from Parkinson's disease as compared to individuals who slept six hours or less.

A study by Diabetes Care suggests that a five-hour or less sleeping time or nine or more hours of sleep each night can possibly increase the risk of developing diabetes. The study also showed that people who slept around seven hours each night had the best chances of survival. And individuals who had less than four and a half hours of sleep had the worst survival rate. Moreover, people who slept nine hours or more also showed higher mortality risk.

What does it all mean? How much sleep do you really need? How much is too much and how much is just enough?

The truth is, when it comes to sleep, there is no magic number. There is no general recommendation because the number of sleep hours shall depend on your age and your activity level. For example, children need to sleep more than adults. But then again, your sleep needs are unique to you. Even people with the same age and activity level may not require the same amount of sleep. It is a case-to-case basis.

According to the National Sleep Foundation, the difference has a lot to do with two factors. And these factors are basal sleep need and sleep debt.

Basal Sleep Need refers to the amount of sleep that an individual requires on a regular basis to achieve optimal performance. Sleep Debt on the other hand, refers to the accumulated sleep individuals lose because of sickness, unhealthy sleep habits and other environmental factors and causes.

According to research studies, to be healthy, adults need a basal sleep of seven to eight hours every night. But when you are having sleeping troubles and you have a high-accumulated sleep debt, it is possible that you still feel exhausted even after sleeping for a full seven to eight hours. People with sleep debt are more likely to feel tired during the mid-afternoon or overnight when the circadian rhythm naturally drops.

The thing is you can pay off a sleep debt by sleeping more every few nights. Then, switch back to your normal basal sleep need when your sleep debt is fully paid.

Get Just the Right Amount of Sleep Each Night

Scientific evidence proves that sleeping too little have detrimental effects on health. It often leads to heart problems, obesity, diabetes, substance abuse, depression and car accidents. But sleeping too much is not healthy either. As a matter of fact, people who get more sleep than they actually need may have higher mortality risks. Depression is also common among people who sleep too much.

In other words, you have to find the middle ground. To be on the safe side and to maximize the benefits of sleep, you should stay within the middle range. And that range is between seven and eight hours. Instead of counting, you can also listen to your body and let it be your guide. Go ahead and get more sleep when you are feeling tired. But get up and sleep less, if you feel like you have already overslept.

Chapter 7 – More Brain Fitness Tips

Can't get enough of brain fitness? Try the following suggestions to boost your brainpower a notch further. They are quite easy and simple, but their impact on brainpower cannot be underestimated.

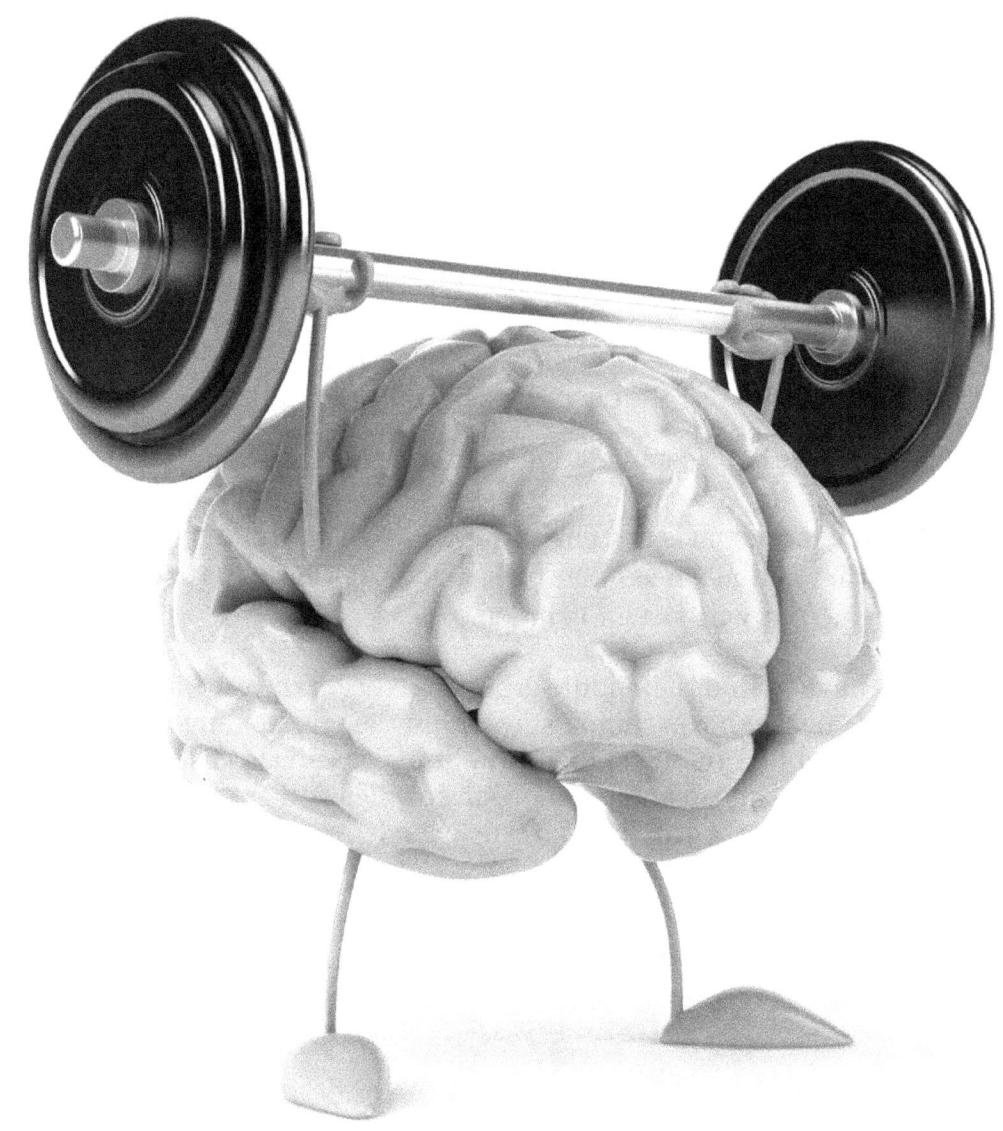

Listen to Music during Your Workout

By listening to music during physical exercise, not only do you get an extra boost of motivation. A research study shows just how helpful this is specifically for cardiovascular rehabilitation patients. Those who put on their jam during exercise demonstrated better performance on verbal fluency tests. Classical music works even better, especially in enhancing spatial processing. It can also improve your linguistic abilities.

Play Golf

You do not have to beat Tiger Woods to exercise the brain. Just take a swing at it. Golf proves to do more than simply work out your arms. Research shows it also leads to structural changes in specific parts of your brain, which are linked to sensory-motor control. That means you can actually get smarter when you hit the green.

Get into Yoga

You may not get better at math in between poses. But studies suggest that yoga helps in improving concentration levels as well as in balancing mood and enhancing cognitive function. It is especially recommended in older adults as yoga also proves to prevent cognitive decline.

Get Organized

A disorganized pile of paper does not only mess up the scene. It also messes up the mind. It is unsightly and it also affects your ability to get some things done. So clear out your space to clear up your mind. In fact, a clean and organized workspace does more than improve productivity. It actually has a direct impact on your cognitive skills and memory.

Doodle

Do not save doodling for the idle time only. Although it seems like a childish exercise, doodling is encouraged during a performance of cognitive tasks. According to one study, it helps enhance memory as it keeps the brain stimulated. So, doodle all you want.

Allow Your Mind to Wander Off

Give your brain a break and just let it wander. Whether you take a stroll down the block or listen to a friend talk endlessly about his or her love life, simply let go and allow your mind to go even in the strangest and most unfamiliar directions. Do not hold your thoughts back. This practice is actually beneficial to cognitive function as it shows to improve problem-solving skills and creativity.

Do Not Forget to Floss

After getting a load of brain foods, do not forget to floss. Flossing does not only take care of your oral health. It also takes care of your brain. How exactly? When plaque accumulates in between your teeth, an immune response is triggered leading to a blockage in the arteries that impede nutrient delivery to the brain. Do not let plaque do this to your brain. Floss because dental is equivalent to mental health.

Mow Your Lawn

Taking care of your green may make your brain sharper. According to one study, lawn mowing helps in the release of chemicals that ease stress and boost memory, especially in older adults.

Write a Pen and Paper than a Keypad

Writing works to stimulate the cells located at the base of the brain. This is called the reticular activating system or RAS, which acts like a filter for all the things the brain needs to process. It prioritizes those that you are currently focused on.

The act of writing wakes the brain up so it pays attention to what you are writing about. Writing with a pen actively engages the brain in the process. If you are trying to study a new language, the learning process is much more effective through note taking with a pen and paper according to studies.

Engage Your Senses

Work on your senses and challenge the brain to keep them sharp. Involve your senses, especially when you are doing routine activities such as eating. For instance, when you are eating hot soup, try closing your eyes so your brain focuses more on the taste and the smell of food rather than merely on how it looks.

Keep Positive Relationships

The people who surround you have more impact on your life than you may realize. They can make you happy or sad. More than that, they can also help you become smarter. According to a study on elderly Americans, positive relationships can assist in protecting against memory loss. So go ahead, sharpen your memory and spend some quality time with your friends and loved ones.

After all, humans are social animals. The Journal of Health and Social Behavior published a recent study that showed people require a variety of brain stimulation. This includes social activities as they help keep the mind sharp. And this benefit manifests later in life as we feel the effects of aging on our memory and neurological processes. According to one study, elderly people who were less active socially are more likely to experience physical and cognitive limitations as compared to those who were more socially active.

Have a Pleasant Conversation

Quick chats can do more than simply pass the time or entertain you. According to studies, socializing enhances cognitive function. Have a simple chat with a friend or colleague. That will help improve your memory and enhance your ability to block distractions. Before working on a big task, have a little talk so you can become more focused on the task at hand a little later.

Laugh Hard, Laugh Often

When you are faced with a tough problem, have a hearty laugh instead of panicking. Research studies suggest that the act of laughing encourages individuals to think in a more creative manner. If you think about it, laughter really is the best medicine.

Remember Your Ancestors

Family means a lot and they mean a lot to brainpower too. According to one study, individuals who had their ancestors in mind before taking cognitive tests recorded better scores than those who thought about something else. Researchers concluded that focusing on family history helps increase sense of control. So, take your time to remember them once in a while. You owe them that much.

Watch SOME TV

A little dose of the tube does not hurt. As a matter of fact, a study shows it may actually help. One study suggests individuals performed better on intelligence tests when they watched a 30-minute TV show as compared to those who worked on puzzles, listened to classical music and read books. According to researchers, some TV time can help individuals relax more than when they engage in other activities. Just make sure you don't overdo it. Keep your TV time to a minimum.

Visualize

Some people are visual learners. If you are one, then it will help a great deal for you to use visual concepts. If you are finding it hard to understand or remember things, try to visualize the information. Take a look at charts, graphics and photographs. Create a mental image of the things you are trying to memorize. And if you could, draw your own graphics. Include them in your notes.

Speak Up

Scientific evidence suggests that people remember ideas better when spoken out loud. Recite it. Speak up and out loud. You may look strange as you talk to yourself, but who cares if it makes you smarter?

Teach.

We have already pointed out that reciting your materials out loud helps with memory. What can improve recall and memory further is teaching. According to psychologists and researchers, teaching a concept to someone else can enhance not only recall, but also your understanding of the material as you make an attempt to explain it to someone else. So when you teach a study partner or a friend, you are not only helping him or her. You are actually doing your brain a favor.

Try It Lying Down

It is important to stand in a proper posture. But according to one study, standing up may not be the most ideal posture after all. The study found that people tend to solve anagrams faster lying down as compared to standing up. Researchers concluded that certain body postures are better at making people more insightful. So, off standing up does not seem to work, try to hang your head lower. You've got nothing to lose.

Drink Plenty of Fluids

The body needs an adequate amount of water to function properly and the brain requires it too. Proper hydration helps a great deal in keeping the brain working properly. Notice that when you are thirsty, you tend to get distracted easily. Moreover, one study showed that individuals who consumed natural fruit and vegetable juices were less likely to have Alzheimer's later on in their lives as compared to people who didn't.

Spice It Up

Spices may not only add more flavors to a dish. Research studies suggest it can help with memory preservation too. Certain spices like cinnamon, sage, cilantro and cumin are known to be great memory boosters. Have some. Sprinkle them over your pasta, salad or shakes.

Drink Coffee

Coffee in the morning may not be so bad after all. It can boost your morning energy and it may also help increase your brainpower. Studies found that an eight-ounce cup of coffee can help enhance attention as well as improve your short-term memory. The key is to keep it at a minimum.

Chew Some Gum

In the middle of a busy day, it is more likely for you to get distracted especially in the mid afternoon. Aside from doing some jumping jacks, you can also chew some gum. It can help make you more alert. More than that, chewing gum can also uplift your mood, so you don't stress out easily.

Have Variety

When you keep doing the same thing every single day, your mind grows idle. The brain gets bored too. So, switch things up and try new activities. Changing up your routine will help stimulate your mind as it encourages the release of dopamine. You will feel more motivated. And a little change in your routine also shows to help with the growth of new neurons.

Read a new book on an unfamiliar topic. Try a new exercise routine. Find something new to do. Go for a hike or play with a ball. Try something else for a change.

Navigate

Do not just rely on GPS to take you around the city. Technology makes things more convenient but doing it yourself can make you smarter. According to one study, navigating cities can improve your spatial memory. London taxi drivers who rely on their mental map of the city showed structural changes in the area of the brain linked to spatial memory.

Learn another Language

It is not only impressive to speak a different language other than your native tongue. It is also helpful with memory. In fact, studies prove that bilingual people are less likely to develop Alzheimer's. It is not too late to learn.

Play an Instrument

It is not just about having a talent to show. It is also about making your brainwork. When you play an instrument the parts of your brain that are responsible for visual-spatial, hearing and motor control become more developed. So, choose your instrument. Play a song you can sing to.

Volunteer

Give back to your community. It feels good. Volunteer work contributes to good health and well-being. In fact, it can help lower stress levels. On top of that, volunteering can also enhance your mental functioning. It is also a great self-esteem booster.

Think Positively

Believe in the power of the brain to get better. Keep challenging yourself. Do not stop learning!

Conclusion

Remember, if we don't use it, we are more likely to lose it!

If you want to stay sharp then make an effort. Keep learning. Choose the right kind of activities that stimulate the brain.

Everybody gets old. And soon enough, we will all experience the consequences of aging. But we can absolutely slow things down.

Stay healthy. Keep your mind and body fit!

You have all the basic information you need about brain fitness. What are you going to do about it? The smart thing to do is to take action now! Go ahead and put everything you've learned to practice!

www.ingramcontent.com/pod-product-compliance
Lightning Source LLC
Chambersburg PA
CBHW081237170526
45165CB00009B/3079